natural healing with aromatherapy

Denise Whichello Brown, BSc.,
Cert. Ed., D.O., M.I.F.P.A., M.I.F.R.

T0352138

British Library Cataloguing in Publication Data: a catalogue record for this title is available from the British Library.

First published in UK 2011 by Hodder Education, part of Hachette UK

Typeset by MPS Limited, a Macmillan Company.

The publisher has used its best endeavours to ensure that the URLs for external websites referred to in this book are correct and active at the time of going to press. However, the publisher and the author have no responsibility for the websites and can make no guarantee that a site will remain live or that the content will remain relevant, decent or appropriate.

Hachette UK's policy is to use papers that are natural, renewable and recyclable products and made from wood grown in sustainable forests. The logging and manufacturing processes are expected to conform to the environmental regulations of the country of origin.

Impression number   10 9 8 7 6 5 4 3 2 1

Year   2015 2014 2013 2012 2011

Contents

Introduction

Aromatherapy has become one of the fastest growing natural healing arts in the UK. It is rapidly gaining respect from orthodox medical practitioners, and qualified clinical aromatherapists now work not only from their own private practices but also in hospitals, hospices and surgeries.

The art of aromatherapy uses pure essential oils which are extracted from various parts of plants and trees. These natural, aromatic, liquid substances, often considered to be the 'life force' or 'soul' of plants, are endowed with a whole host of therapeutic properties. They are remarkably versatile and may be used in various ways. This book aims to show you how to use essential oils safely and effectively on your friends and family without creating harmful side-effects, unlike many chemical drugs.

Aromatherapy is a holistic therapy which can be used to promote physical, mental and spiritual health equilibrium. It forms part of a holistic healing regime which involves searching for the root causes of an illness, rather than its symptoms, and awakening the body's innate ability to heal itself, leading to a state of balance. Aromatherapy involves far more than the application of essential oils. To achieve 'whole healing', factors such as diet and lifestyle must always be considered.

Since I have stepped into the world of essential oils, my life has been completely transformed. I do hope that you will allow aromatherapy to become part of your daily life and that this book will encourage you to learn more about these fascinating, healing, essential oils which can help you to achieve balance of mind, body and spirit.

1

buying and caring for essential oils and how to use them

In this chapter you will find out how to identify high quality pure essential oils; the purity of your essential oils is important if you wish to achieve the best results. You also need to know how to care for and store your precious essential oils and aromatherapy blends.

There are so many ways in which essential oils can be used for health and healing. You can use them in your bath or shower to combat stress, or to rejuvenate you at the end of a long hard day. Find out how to make a footbath for feel-good feet or a hand bath to soothe painful hands. Learn how to make a compress or a gargle, how to use essential oils in an inhalation or an oil burner, and how to make up aromatherapy blends for massage. Bring the healing art of aromatherapy into your daily life!

Quality and adulteration

It is vital to use only high-quality pure essential oils for optimum results. It is most unfortunate that many essential oils available on the market today are of poor quality and, therefore, cannot help alleviate health problems. Only five per cent of all essential oils produced in the world are used for aromatherapy. Essential oil traders supply mostly to the perfume, food, pharmaceutical and chemical manufacturing industries. Suppliers of essential oils will sometimes adulterate their oils by adding synthetic ingredients, alcohols, vegetable oil, cheap chemical constituents or low-cost essential oils. They may even substitute an entire essential oil with a cheaper, similar oil for commercial gain (e.g. lavendin may be sold as lavender).

Essential oils used in aromatherapy must, of course, be as pure, natural and 'whole' as possible if they are to have the desired therapeutic effects. Synthetic materials which simulate the aroma and appearance of an essential oil cannot have the same therapeutic properties as an essential oil and should not be used in therapy. Synthetic chemicals also carry the risk of harmful and unpleasant side-effects, as do synthetic drugs. If oils are referred to as 'nature identical' this implies that the oil is synthetic and produced in the laboratory and is, therefore, unsuitable for aromatherapy. Synthetic oils also do not possess the 'vital force' or 'life force' of essential oils which comes from living plants. Nor do chemicals contain the 'vibration' of natural living plants.

Since most aromatherapy suppliers buy essential oils from importers who supply the perfume and food industries it is important to seek a supplier who deals mainly with essential oils intended only for therapeutic use.

Care and storage

Essential oils are extremely precious and should be treated with respect – they can also be very expensive. They are damaged by ultraviolet light and deteriorate more rapidly at the blue end of the spectrum than the red. Therefore, essential oils should be stored in amber-coloured bottles (if you do keep your essential oils in blue bottles then they should be kept in the dark – this is less important if your bottles are brown).

Essential oils should never be placed in direct sunlight so avoid sunny windowsills or shelves on radiators – no matter how attractive the bottles look! Essential oils do not like extremes of temperatures. They are highly volatile, which means that they evaporate rapidly. Always replace the caps immediately and ensure that the tops are tightly closed when the oils are not in use. Essential oils must be cared for properly to prevent chemical degradation (i.e. a process whereby the quality of the essential oil is reduced over time) which will occur with prolonged storage and poor storage conditions.

Pure essential oils will last for approximately three years from the bottling date. In excellent storage conditions (i.e. amber bottles in a cool place with no air space) they will keep for about five years. Citrus oils tend to have a shorter shelf life.

Once essential oils have been diluted in a carrier oil, the shelf life reduces dramatically. For maximum benefit use freshly made-up blends. A blend will keep for about three to six months if it is stored in an amber-coloured bottle in a cool place away from sunlight.

Dos and don'ts of buying and storage

* Clear glass or plastic bottles do not contain pure essential oils. Always buy oils in amber-coloured bottles.
* How old are the essential oils? When were they bottled?
* Are the oils in direct sunlight?
* Are the essential oils all the same price? If they are, then you are definitely not purchasing pure essential oils. For instance, pure essential oil of rose will be far more expensive than lavender or rosemary.
* Have the essential oils been diluted with any carrier oils? If so, when were they blended?

* Have the essential oils been adulterated with synthetic materials or bulking agents?
* Does the aromatherapy trader deal mostly with the perfume and food industries? Always look for an aromatherapy specialist.
* Does your supplier know about the essential oils?
* If blends are being sold, is there a qualified aromatherapist on the staff?
* Has the supplier been recommended to you?
* How long has the aromatherapy firm been established?
* Essential oils should always be kept away from young children. If they are taken internally some essential oils can be highly dangerous.
* Never leave bottled pure essential oils standing on plastic, polished or painted surfaces which can be damaged by the chemical constituents.
* Always store essential oils away from naked flames.
* Store essential oils away from your homoeopathic medications which may be antidoted by the more powerful aromas.

Two tips for checking for the purity of essential oils:
1 Put one drop of pure essential oil on a piece of paper and see if it leaves a greasy mark. If your essential oil is pure then there should be no greasy mark. Despite their name essential oils are not oily.
2 Rub a little essential oil between your thumb and index finger. Does it have a greasy feel? If it does then the oil has been adulterated.

Using essential oils

There are numerous ways in which essential oils can be used. I will outline some of the easiest and most effective techniques, but I urge you to be creative and fill your home with essential oils. You can create a beautiful aromatic environment while preventing or healing a multitude of common disorders.

External use

Baths

Aromatherapy baths have been employed for pleasure and therapeutic purposes throughout history. The Greek physician Hippocrates, the Father of Medicine, claimed that 'the way to health is to have an aromatic bath and a scented massage daily'.

Baths were particularly enjoyed by the ancient Egyptians, who had public baths, as did the Romans, for whom baths were an important aspect of social life. Water itself is therapeutic: 'water cures' are advocated by naturopaths, and various forms of hydrotherapy can be found in use nowadays at health farms and natural therapy centres. Baths are an effective way of using essential oils as the oils act in two ways: by absorption into the skin and by inhalation.

Essential oils are simple to use in the bath. Just fill the bath and sprinkle about six drops of your chosen undiluted oil into the water, agitating it thoroughly. Do not add the essential oil until you have run the bath completely, otherwise the oil will evaporate with the heat of the water and the therapeutic properties will be lost before you climb in! Always disperse the oil – if you inadvertently sit down on neat essential oil of, say, tangerine you will jump up again very quickly! Shut the door to keep the precious aromas in and stay in the bath for at least 15 minutes to allow the oil to penetrate deeply into your body tissues.

As essential oils are not soluble in water you may blend your six drops of essential oil with a teaspoon of carrier oil for a moisturizing bath. This is particularly beneficial for those with dry skin. Choose any vegetable oil such as sweet almond, avocado or jojoba. You could mix up enough oil for several baths. Your skin will feel soft, nourished and supple.

I would strongly advise anyone with a sensitive skin to *always* blend the essential oil with a carrier oil. Also, when using essential oils in a bath for babies and young children the oils should always be blended with a carrier oil. Undiluted essential oils can damage the eyes and babies and toddlers do have a tendency to rub their eyes.

Use one drop in a baby's bath and two drops in a toddler's bath diluted in a teaspoon of a carrier oil such as sweet almond oil. I can endorse the effectiveness of this method.

Any essential oil may be added to a bath. However, caution should be exercised with the citrus oils and the stronger essences such as black pepper and peppermint if you have particularly sensitive skin. Just add three drops instead of six.

Footbaths and hand baths

Footbaths and hand baths are highly beneficial in situations where it is impractical to enjoy a full aromatherapy bath – perhaps if you are elderly or have a disability. Footbaths, in particular, are incredibly relaxing at the end of a long, hard day especially when you feel too lethargic to undress. They are excellent for foot conditions such as athlete's foot and pain and swelling in the feet. Hand baths help to relieve the pain, stiffness and swelling of arthritis. Anyone who uses their hands extensively, such as hairdressers, gardeners or those working with computers, should have regular hand baths.

Add six drops of essential oil to a bowl of hand-hot water just before you immerse your feet or hands and soak for about ten to fifteen minutes. If you wish you may mix your essential oils with a carrier oil.

There is no excuse for not having time for aromatherapy. Enjoy a footbath while you are reading or studying and a hand or footbath while watching your favourite television programme. Remember to use six drops.

Sitz baths and bidets

A sitz bath is beneficial in cases of cystitis, haemorrhoids, vaginal discharge, stitches after childbirth and so on. Sprinkle about four to six drops of pure essential oil into a bowl of hand-hot water and sit in the bowl for about ten minutes. Your essential oils may be added to a carrier oil. If you have a bidet then use the same number of drops. Ensure that the essential oil and water are thoroughly mixed.

Showers

A shower can never be as relaxing as a bath when using essential oils. However, it can be quite a stimulating way to begin your day.

Apply six drops of essential oil to a sponge or a flannel and rub all over your body towards the end of your shower. Alternatively, add six drops of essential oil to two teaspoons of carrier oil and apply to your body before stepping into the shower. Make sure that you inhale the warming vapours. Another method is to plug the tray of your shower, turn on the water and add six drops of essential oil to the water. You will absorb the oils through your feet and as the vapours rise you will inhale them.

Some essential oil suppliers stock shower gel to which essential oils may be added.

Compresses

Compresses can be used for a variety of disorders such as muscular aches and pains, bruises, rheumatic and arthritic pain, headaches and sprains. They are a very effective way of relieving pain and reducing inflammation and swelling.

You may apply compresses either hot or cold. Alternate hot and cold compresses are valuable for treating sprains. As a general rule, where there is fever, acute pain or hot swellings use a cold compress. When treating chronic (long-term) pain use a hot compress.

To make a compress, mix approximately six drops of essential oil into a small bowl of hot or cold water. Soak any piece of absorbent material such as a flannel, handkerchief, piece of sheeting or towelling in the solution ensuring that as much essential oil as possible is absorbed by your fabric. Squeeze out the compress so it does not drip everywhere and apply to the affected area. Wrap clingfilm around it or secure with a bandage. Leave for about two hours or even overnight. Where there is a fever replace with a new cold compress when necessary.

Gargles and mouthwashes

Gargles are particularly beneficial for sore throats, respiratory problems, loss of voice and halitosis (bad breath). After dental surgery gargling can help to relieve pains and inflammation, reduce blood flow and speed up the healing process. Gargle twice daily, although if the problem is acute then you can gargle every two hours.

Put two drops of essential oil into half a glass of water. Stir well, gargle and spit it out. Do not swallow. Stir again and repeat. You may also use one to two teaspoons of organic cider vinegar or lemon and/or a teaspoon of honey in your gargle. Honey has anti-inflammatory and antibacterial properties and is renowned for its soothing action on the throat, and fresh lemon juice is antibacterial, detoxifying and counteracts acidity. Antiseptic oils such as tea tree, lemon and thyme are excellent for treating sore throats. German/Roman chamomile, geranium and sandalwood will also soothe inflammation. Myrrh and tea tree combined is very useful for treating mouth ulcers.

Inhalations

Inhalation of essential oils works upon the body, mind and spirit.

On a physical level there is a strong action on the mucous membranes of the nose, the lungs and the respiratory system in general. Conditions such as asthma, bronchitis, catarrh, coughs, colds, sinusitis and sore throats can all benefit enormously.

The inhalation of essential oils has a profound effect on the nervous system, helping to relieve insomnia, anxiety and stress-related disorders and lifting depression and negativity.

On a spiritual level some essential oils such as frankincense, cedarwood and linden blossom raise the consciousness and provide an excellent aid for meditation.

Steam inhalation

Add three drops of essential oil to a bowl of hot water. Cover your head with a towel and lean over the bowl inhaling deeply for a few minutes. Keep your eyes closed to avoid irritation. If someone who has asthma uses this method then just one drop is adequate. Take care with the hot water if there are small children around.

Handkerchief/tissue

Sprinkle a few drops of essential oil on to a handkerchief, paper towel or tissue and take a few deep breaths. This method is particularly effective for relieving nasal congestion (use cajeput, eucalyptus) and also for stopping panic attacks (use lavender). Place the handkerchief in your pocket and you can continue to inhale the aroma throughout the day. Sufferers of motion sickness will also find this method effective.

Hands

In a crisis situation put one drop of lavender on to your palm, rub your hands together, cup them over your nose and then breathe deeply. Avoid the eye area and ensure that your eyes are closed.

Room spray

A room spray is an excellent way of purifying the atmosphere. Pour 250 ml of water into a plant spray and add 15–20 drops of essential oil. Shake the bottle well and spray the room. You can even spray carpets and curtains. Do not spray on to polished surfaces.

Sprays can also be used to relieve irritation and pain as in chickenpox, shingles, burns and any infectious skin diseases.

Vaporizers

For home use, I recommend a clay vaporizer heated by a night light. These are readily available. Put a few teaspoons of water into the loose bowl on top and sprinkle about six drops of essential oil into it. Light the night light and the oil will diffuse into the air.

For relaxation burn oils such as lavender, chamomile, sandalwood or ylang ylang.

For meditation try frankincense.

To repel insects use citronella.

Pillow and nightwear method

Place a few drops of essential oil on to a pillow or your nightwear for relief from insomnia and to encourage easier and deeper breathing. If desired, you could put the drops on to a piece of cotton wool and place it inside the pillow case. Lavender and chamomile are both excellent.

Candles

Add one to two drops of essential oil to the warm wax of a candle, taking care to avoid the wick since essential oils are flammable.

Massage

Massage, even without essential oils, is a powerful therapy. The combination of pure essential oils and massage is especially potent. Massage is one of the most effective and beneficial treatment techniques. Essential oil constituents pass through the skin and into the bloodstream and can be carried to all the cells of the body.

Essential oils are not usually applied in an undiluted form to the skin except for emergencies such as burns, cuts or a sting. They must be blended with a suitable carrier oil in the appropriate dilution. When blending essential oil with a base oil, the essential oil content is usually between one per cent and three per cent. A massage takes between 10 ml and 20 ml of oil. Since a teaspoon holds approximately 5 ml, a treatment will require only two to four teaspoons of base oil.

The following guidelines will help you to blend your oils in the appropriate dilutions.

* 3 drops of essential oil to 10 ml of carrier oil
* 4–5 drops of essential oil to 15 ml of carrier oil
* 6 drops of essential oil to 20 ml of carrier oil
* 15 drops of essential oil to 50 ml of carrier oil
* 30 drops of essential oil to 100 ml of carrier oil

Oils which have been blended should be stored in amber-coloured bottles just like pure essential oils. If you wish to blend your essential oils into a vegetable-based lotion, rather than an oil, the dilution will be the same. Always label your bottles with the date and the oils that you have selected. When blending essential oils and base oils it is important to bear in mind that an increased concentration of essential oil does not imply that the formula will be more effective. Excessive amounts of essential oil may create unpleasant side-effects and reactions. I would not advise you to put more than five essential oils together in one blend – usually two or three will be quite sufficient to create the desired therapeutic effects.

It is important to consider both the physical and emotional problems of the recipient of the treatment. Since many physical ailments stem from an emotional source, I strongly recommend the selection of at least one oil for any emotional imbalances. Remember that you are treating the whole person rather than the symptoms.

Always allow the recipient to smell the aromatic formula before you start the treatment. Rub a small amount on to the back of the recipient's hand. If the aroma is pleasurable then it will have a beneficial effect.

2

carrier oils

Pure essential oils are highly concentrated and therefore should not be used undiluted on the skin. Instead they are blended with a carrier oil, which is also known as a 'base' or 'fixed' oil.

It is important to use high quality carrier oils for optimum results. You should choose cold-pressed, unrefined and additive-free carrier oils wherever possible. Other factors that you should bear in mind are the texture, absorbability and the aroma of the base oil.

Four of the most commonly used carrier oils are sweet almond, apricot kernel, peach kernel and grapeseed. These carrier oils can be used on their own, but may also be blended with small amounts of thicker, more viscous and more expensive carrier oils such as avocado, calendula or evening primrose, which are also explored in this chapter.

Have fun with your carrier oils and why not formulate your own personal blend!

Essential oils are highly concentrated in their pure state and they should not be used undiluted directly on the skin. Therefore, a natural medium is required for an aromatherapy massage treatment and is referred to as the carrier, base or fixed oil. Since the carrier oil constitutes a large proportion of an aromatherapy blend its quality should be given careful consideration. Carrier oils as well as essential oils should be of the highest quality if maximum therapeutic benefits are to be obtained.

The carrier oil chosen should be cold pressed. In the process of cold pressing the use of excessive heat is avoided and therefore any changes to the natural characteristics of the oil are minimized. Oils produced by the process of 'hot extraction', although much cheaper, are unsuitable for use in aromatherapy as they are of an inferior quality.

The base oil should also be unrefined and untreated by chemicals. The process of refining includes the removal of colour by bleaching, removing taste and smell, extracting natural fatty acids, which can lead to cloudiness, and the removal of free fatty acids.

Vegetable oils have therapeutic properties in their own right and contain many vitamins and minerals, but the more highly processed the vegetable oils are, the less vitamin content will be retained. Colour, other additives and synthetic antioxidants to extend the shelf life may also be added at the oil pressing factories, which is also undesirable. For the purpose of aromatherapy always use cold pressed (preferably the 'virgin' type which is the first oil to be collected), unrefined, additive-free carrier oils. It is highly unlikely that you will find these oils on the shelves of your supermarket! Since the carrier oil is by far the largest part of any massage blend, always choose it carefully.

Mineral oil (purified, light petroleum oil), such as commercial baby oil, should never be used in aromatherapy as a carrier oil. Mineral oils tend to clog the pores whereas some of the vegetable oil molecules are absorbed through the skin. Mineral oils also do not have the nutritional constituents (vitamins, minerals and fatty acids) of the vegetable oils which nourish and benefit the skin.

Mineral oil is used by the cosmetics industry because it does not become rancid. However, it stays on the skin like an 'oil slick' and prevents it from breathing.

The shelf life of a base oil is dependent upon its fatty acid and vitamin E content. Vegetable oils which have a high proportion of saturated fatty acids will keep longer than those which are high in unsaturated fatty acids. The presence of vitamin E in the carrier oil will also increase the shelf life.

There is a wide variety of vegetable oils suitable for aromatherapy massage. Some of the most commonly used carrier oils include sweet almond, apricot kernel, peach kernel and grapeseed. These oils are not too thick and have hardly any smell and so will not mask the aroma of the essential oils. Some aromatherapists will use these carrier oils on their own but many prefer to add other thicker, more viscous oils to their aromatherapy blends, such as avocado, jojoba and evening primrose oil. My own particular special blend includes sweet almond, apricot and peach kernel, jojoba, avocado, calendula and wheatgerm.

When choosing a carrier oil factors to bear in mind include:
* quality (choose a cold-pressed, unrefined, additive-free oil)
* texture (thick, sticky oils do NOT make a good massage medium)
* absorbability (choose a vegetable and NOT a mineral oil)
* aroma (a strong smell will mask the aroma of the essential oils).

The following section lists and describes the principal properties and indications of a range of carrier oils. Please note that some carrier oils are used on their own, or they may be blended with the thicker, more viscous carrier oils.

Almond oil (sweet)

Latin name: *Prunus amygdalis* var. *dulcis*
Family: *Rosaceae*

Sweet almond oil is one of the most widely used carrier oils in aromatherapy since it is low in odour and is not too thick, sticky or heavy. It is easily absorbed by the skin and is highly recommended for aromamassage.

The fruits of the almond tree look like a small green apricot and the best quality oil, which is extracted by cold pressing the kernels, is pale yellow in colour. It has a delicate, rather sweet smell and is rich in vitamins and unsaturated fatty acids. If the oil is refined and chemically extracted it is cheaper due to the higher yield but such oil is not really suitable for aromatherapy.

Uses:
- * beneficial for all skin types
- * an excellent emollient for nourishing the skin
- * helps to relieve itching induced by conditions such as eczema, psoriasis and dermatitis
- * soothes inflammation
- * nourishes dry and prematurely aged skin
- * suitable for sensitive skin
- * soothes sunburn
- * excellent for moisturizing dry hair that has been chemically treated or exposed to too much sun.

Sweet almond oil is highly recommended and may be used as a base oil up to 100 per cent.

Special precautions:
Sweet almond oil is considered to be a very safe carrier oil.

Apricot kernel oil

Latin name: *Prunus armeniaca*
Family: *Rosaceae*

Apricot kernel oil is very similar to sweet almond oil although it is more expensive as it is produced in smaller quantities.

The oil is obtained by cold pressing the kernels and contains vitamins and unsaturated fatty acids.

Apricot kernel oil is used in many cosmetic products, such as in facial scrubs and masks, to clear away dead skin cells, as well as in soaps, shampoos and creams.

The oil is pale yellow and has a stronger odour than sweet almond – rather marzipan-like. Apricot kernel oil has a wonderful silky texture and is easily absorbed by the skin. It is a most delightful carrier oil to use in an aromamassage.

Uses:
* excellent for all skin types
* nourishes dry skin
* relieves itching and therefore helps conditions such as eczema
* beneficial for sensitive and prematurely aged skin.

Apricot kernel oil may be used as a base 100 per cent although it is usually added to a blend due to its enriching and nourishing properties. It is an excellent choice for a facial oil.

Special precautions:
Apricot kernel oil is completely safe with no reported toxic effects. Interestingly, however, ingestion of apricot kernels is the most common form of cyanide poisoning – so avoid eating them!

Avocado oil

Latin name: *Persea americana*
Family: *Lauraceae*

This wonderful dark rich green carrier oil is cold pressed from the dried flesh of avocado pears which have been damaged and therefore are not of a high enough quality for marketing.

It has a distinctive aroma similar to the ripe fruit. Avocado oil is rich in lecithin, vitamins A, B and D and minerals as well as saturated and unsaturated fatty acids. It has a long shelf life.

Uses:
* moisturizes and softens all types of skin
* beneficial for dry, dehydrated skin as it is such a highly penetrative oil
* soothes skin inflammation
* prevents premature ageing

* helps to heal the skin
* may help poor circulation
* maintains the suppleness and elasticity of the skin
* offers some protection from the sun and is sometimes mixed with sesame oil for this purpose.

Avocado oil is usually added to a blend in up to a 10 per cent dilution.

Special precautions:

A very safe oil which does not cause sensitization, but do not use the colourless, refined, bleached oil.

Calendula oil (also known as marigold oil)

Latin name: *Calendula officinalis*
Family: *Asteraceae* (or *Compositae*)

Calendula oil is a macerated oil which means that the wonderful yellow or bright orange flowers are macerated in a fixed oil to produce the orange-yellow coloured calendula oil.

Uses:
* renowned for all skin disorders
* soothes inflammation
* heals chapped and cracked skin
* useful for varicose veins and broken veins
* relieves itching and skin conditions such as eczema
* helps to reduce thread veins on the face
* soothes and heals cracked nipples
* reduces and prevents scarring
* useful for bruises
* soothes burns
* makes a wonderful addition to hand and foot creams.

Calendula oil would normally be added to your basic carrier oil in up to a 10 per cent dilution, although it may be used in its own right on specific areas.

Special precautions:

Calendula oil has no known side-effects.

Evening primrose oil

Latin name: *Oenothera biennis*
Family: *Onagraceae*

The oil is cold pressed from the seeds and is rich in linoleic acid (approximately 70 per cent), which is in a polyunsaturated fatty acid, and also contains GLA (gamma linoleic acid), which is also present in borage oil.

Heralded as a 'miracle of modern times' it has become increasingly popular to take evening primrose oil internally in capsules for a whole host of conditions.

Uses:
* excellent for dry skin
* ideal for sensitive and allergic-type skin
* calms down redness and inflammation
* counteracts premature ageing of the skin and wrinkles
* favourable for skin conditions aggravated by hormonal imbalances, e.g. acne and puberty, prior to menstruation and during the menopause
* may improve varicose veins
* beneficial for dry hair and dandruff.

Evening primrose oil is usually added to a blend in up to a 10 per cent dilution.

Special precautions:
Evening primrose oil is a very safe oil when used externally.

Grapeseed oil

Latin name: *Vitis vinifera*
Family: *Vitaceae*

Unfortunately it is not available cold pressed (and cold-pressed, unrefined oils are the finest oils for aromatherapy). However, it is a very popular oil for massage and aromatherapy as it is a very smooth oil which is not greasy and is also colourless and odourless. It contains a high percentage of linoleic acid and also vitamin E.

Uses:

* may be used on all skin types
* easily absorbed by the skin.

Grapeseed oil can be used as a base oil 100 per cent.

Special precautions:

It is a very safe oil with no known contraindications.

Jojoba oil

Latin name: *Simmondsia chinensis/Simmondsia sinensis*
Family: *Buxaceae*

It is a golden oil which is very stable and as it does not oxidize it does not become rancid and has a very long shelf life. If jojoba oil is left in a very cold place it will solidify, but will very rapidly liquefy when brought back to room temperature. It has a faint, slightly sweet aroma and a wonderful texture. Jojoba is used in creams, lotions and lipsticks.

Uses:

* combats inflammation and therefore is useful for arthritis, dermatitis and swellings of all descriptions
* suitable for all types of skin
* nourishes and moisturizes dry skin
* combats the drying effects of the sun
* helps to heal wounds
* beneficial for chapped skin and nappy rash
* prevents the build-up of sebum and therefore useful for oily skin
* relieves itchy skin conditions such as eczema and psoriasis
* helps control acne
* conditions, protects and renews the hair.

Jojoba is usually added in up to a 10 per cent dilution as it is more expensive than some other base oils. However, it may be used 100 per cent on small areas.

Jojoba makes a wonderful facial oil which can be compared favourably with any expensive cream.

Blend jojoba with essential oils such as rose, frankincense, neroli and carrot seed to prevent and reduce the signs of ageing.

Special precautions:

A safe carrier oil which I have never seen any reactions to but allergic reactions have been rarely reported.

Peach kernel oil

Latin name: *Prunus persica*
Family: *Rosaceae*

Peach kernel oil is very similar to apricot kernel oil and sweet almond oil. It is extracted by cold pressing the kernels if it is a high quality oil and is made up mostly of unsaturated fatty acids including linoleic acid. It is pale yellow in colour and virtually odourless with a light texture which makes it a wonderful carrier oil for aromatherapy.

Uses:
* an effective moisturizer for dry, dehydrated skin
* relieves itching as in eczema and psoriasis
* beneficial for mature skin
* suitable for dry, damaged or coloured hair
* good for sensitive skin.

Peach kernel oil may be used as a base 100 per cent although it is usually added to a blend in a dilution of approximately 10 per cent.

Special precautions:

Peach kernel oil is totally safe with no reported side-effects.

3

A–Z of essential oils

There is a vast array of essential oils to choose from. It is not necessary to buy an extensive range for use at home on friends and family. A few essential oils are all you need to meet your everyday requirements, and will treat a wide range of common ailments. Begin with bergamot, chamomile, cypress, eucalyptus, geranium, lavender, lemon, peppermint and rosemary. You can then gradually increase your collection.

Every essential oil has a profile, showing how it works upon the body and mind, as well as the spirit. Keywords are included which indicate at a glance the primary effects of each essential oil. Don't forget that certain precautions may need to be observed before you use some essential oils.

Basil (French)/sweet basil/common basil

Latin name: *Ocimum basilicum*
Family: *Lamiaceae* (or *Labiatae*)

Principal properties and indications – keywords

* Awakening
* Clarifying
* Decongestive
* Stimulating
* Strengthening
* Uplifting

Digestive system

* Recommended for digestive disorders.

Genito-urinary system

* Recommended for delayed menstruation, scanty periods and menstrual cramps.

Muscles/joints

* Relieves muscle spasms, cramp, gout, arthritis and rheumatism.
* Use after exercise for tired muscles.

Nervous system

* Probably one of the best nerve tonics as basil uplifts, clarifies, strengthens and restores.
* Use for mental fatigue and inability to concentrate as it is reputed to clear the head.
* Relieves nervous tension, depression and nervous exhaustion.

Respiratory system

* All respiratory problems including asthma, bronchitis, coughs, colds and whooping cough.
* Excellent for clearing the head.
* Use for catarrh, earache, nasal polyps, rhinitis, sinusitis, head colds, headaches and migraines.

Effects on spirit

* Uplifts and awakens the spirit, encouraging the development of intuition.

Special precautions

* Take care in pregnancy (although toxicity is unproven).
* Use in low dilution with sensitive skin (although sensitivity is rare).
* Do not use Exotic basil, also known as Comoran or Reunion basil.

Use basil as an inhalant to clear away catarrh and sinusitis. Basil is an excellent oil for clearing the head and it aids concentration and focuses the mind. Burn it to help you study!

Benzoin

Latin name: *Styrax benzoin*
Family: *Styraceae*

Principal properties and indications – keywords

* Comforting
* Soothing
* Gets things moving
* Warming
* Healing

Circulatory system

* Stimulates the circulation.
* Warms and regulates the heart.

Genito-urinary system

* Relieves all vaginal infections, discharges and irritations such as cystitis.
* Reduces fluid retention.

Muscles/joints

* Combats arthritis, gout, rheumatism and fibrositis.

Nervous system

* A warming oil that beings comfort to the recently bereaved and sad, lonely or depressed individuals.

Respiratory system

* Benzoin is a component of Friar's Balsam and is valuable for respiratory problems such as asthma, bronchitis, colds, coughs, flu, laryngitis and throat infections.

Skin
* Excellent for cracked and chapped skin.
* Soothes redness, irritation and dermatitis and encourages healing of sores and wounds.

Effects on spirit
* Protects the spirit. Uplifting and beneficial for the heart and solar plexus.

Special precautions
* Do not take internally (it is not a distilled oil).

Benzoin is a very useful addition to any foot or hand cream. It soothes redness and irritation and prevents and treats cracked and chapped hands and feet.

Bergamot

Latin name: *Citrus bergamia*
Family: *Rutaceae*

Principal properties and indications – keywords
* Antidepressant
* Antiseptic
* Balancing
* Uplifting

Digestive system
* A tonic for the digestion stimulating a poor appetite and alleviating gas, colic and indigestion.
* Relieves halitosis (bad breath) when used as a gargle.
* Recommended for eating disorders such as anorexia and bulimia.

Genito-urinary system
* Has a strong affinity for this system helping cystitis, vaginal discharges, thrush and pruritis (itching) – use in the early stages for maximum benefit.

Nervous system
* Sedative yet uplifting.
* Ideal for all states of anxiety, depression and stress-related conditions.

Respiratory system
* Relieves sore throats, tonsillitis, colds, flu and all respiratory infections.

Skin
* Improves all stress-related skin conditions such as eczema and psoriasis.
* Use for contagious conditions such as scabies, chickenpox and head lice.
* Helps oily skin, acne, spots, boils and herpes.
* Effective for cold sores, chickenpox and shingles.

Effects on spirit
* Uplifts and refreshes the spirit encouraging a joyful approach to life.

Special precautions
* Do not apply prior to sunbathing as it increases the photosensitivity of the skin due to its bergaptene content, which accelerates tanning.

Bergamot is a very uplifting oil and is renowned for its ability to treat anxiety and all stress-related disorders. A great oil to put in your bath or burn when you're feeling low.

Black pepper
Latin name: *Piper nigrum*
Family: *Piperaceae*

Principal properties and indications – keywords
* Detoxifying
* Eliminative
* 'Get-up-and-go'
* Restorative
* Stimulant
* Tonic
* Warming

Circulatory system
* A warming oil excellent for poor circulation.
* Recommended for anaemia and after heavy bleeding.
* Helpful for chilblains.

Digestive system
* Dispels toxins from the digestive system alleviating colic, constipation and food poisoning.
* Stimulates a poor appetite.
* Restores tone to the colon.

Muscles/joints
* Restores tone to the skeletal system.
* Relieves muscular aches and pains, neuralgia, stiffness, arthritis, rheumatism, sprains and strains.
* Recommended prior to training to improve performance and afterwards to prevent pain and stiffness.

Nervous system
* Stimulates the mind, aiding concentration and strengthening the nerves.
* Useful for coldness, indifference and apathy.

Respiratory system
* Drives out coughs, colds, chills, catarrh and phlegm.

Effects on spirit
* A grounding oil which also encourages change and instils positive thoughts and actions.

Special precautions
* None.

A great 'get-up-and-go' oil that strengthens the nerves, combats apathy and fills you with courage and stamina.

Cajeput
Latin name: *Melaleuca leucadendron/cajeputi*
Family: *Myrtaceae*

Principal properties and indications – keywords
* Antiseptic
* Decongestive
* Penetrating
* Stimulating
* Warming

Digestive system

* Helpful for gastric spasms, upset stomachs and diarrhoea.

Genito-urinary system

* Alleviates all urinary infections such as cystitis and urethritis.

Muscles/joints

* Excellent for pain relief.
* Use for all aches, painful joints, arthritis, rheumatism, gout, sciatica, sprains and strains.
* Recommended for sports injuries.

Nervous system

* Clears and stimulates the mind and aids concentration.

Respiratory system

* Valuable for the respiratory system as an inhalant and a chest rub.
* Encourages the expulsion of mucus.
* Useful as a gargle for laryngitis and throat infections.
* Excellent as an inhalation for sinusitis and catarrh.

Skin

* Useful for oily skin, spots, boils and head lice.

Effects on spirit

* Elevates the spirit and encourages the creation of new pathways.

Special precautions

* Take care with sensitive skin (although irritation unproven).
* Use in a low dilution.

My favourite decongestant which has a gentler action than the more commonly used eucalyptus oil. Use the inhalation method to loosen mucus and use cajeput in a chest rub for coughs and colds.

Carrot seed

Latin name: *Daucus carota*
Family: *Umbelliferae* (or *Apiaceae*)

Principal properties and indications – keywords

* Detoxifying
* Revitalizing
* Stimulating
* Tonic

Circulatory system

* Stimulates poor circulation and purifies and detoxifies blood and lymph.
* Helpful for anaemia.
* Boosts the immune system.

Digestive system

* Alleviates constipation, irritable bowel syndrome, flatulence and liver problems.
* Useful for eating disorders such as anorexia.

Genito-urinary system

* Combats fluid retention and cystitis.
* Regulates the menstrual cycle and balances the hormones.

Nervous system

* Recommended for confusion and indecision – it enables us to see situations more clearly.
* Stimulating and revitalizing.

Skin

* Useful for skin problems, it is a tonic increasing the elasticity of the skin.
* Ideal for mature skins.
* Reduces scarring, for instance after acne.
* Revitalizes tired, dull, lifeless skin.

Effects on spirit

* Strengthens inner vision.

Special precautions

* None.

Add three drops to 10 ml carrier oil or 10 g cream to create a wonderful moisturiser to prevent and reduce wrinkling.

Chamomile, Roman

Latin name: *Anthemis nobilis/Chamaemelum nobile*
Family: *Asteraceae* (or *Compositae*)

Principal properties and indications – keywords
* Anti-inflammatory
* Calming
* Children
* Sedative

Circulatory system
* Useful for boosting the immune system and reducing susceptibility to infection.
* Indicated for anaemia.

Digestive system
* Calms the digestive system easing gas and colic.
* Excellent for children's digestive problems.
* Eases inflammation in the bowels and thus important for IBS (irritable bowel syndrome).
* Useful for the liver and gall bladder.

Genito-urinary system
* Ideal for the menopause and PMS.
* Balances the menstrual cycle.
* Helpful for painful and scanty menstruation.

Muscular/joints
* Useful for inflamed joints and tendons.
* Relieves pain.
* Beneficial for gout.
* Combats headaches, migraine and neuralgia.
* Relaxes muscles, especially when associated with nervous tension.

Nervous system
* Exerts a pronounced calming effect on the nervous system and mind.
* Ideal for oversensitive individuals.
* Soothes restlessness, irritability and impatience.
* Useful for insomnia.

Skin

* Beneficial for all types of skin including sensitive, red and dry skin.
* Suitable for eczema and psoriasis.
* Soothes irritated and inflamed skin.
* Useful for cracked nipples.
* Recommended after shaving.

Effects on spirit

* Promotes a harmonious, peaceful and joyful spirit.

Special precautions

* None. A safe oil, suitable for babies, young children and highly sensitive individuals.

A must-have oil for babies and children. Chamomile eases colic, soothes restlessness and temper tantrums and promotes a good night's sleep.

Citronella

Latin name: *Cymbopogon nardus*
Family: *Poaceae* (or *Gramineae*)

Principal properties and indications – keywords

* Clearing
* Insect repellent
* Refreshing
* Stimulating

Digestive system

* Helpful for poor and sluggish digestion.
* Combats candida.

Genito-urinary system

* Useful for fluid retention.

Nervous system

* Banishes extreme fatigue, lethargy and exhaustion.
* Clears the mind.

Respiratory system

* Helpful for colds and flu.

Skin

* Refreshes sweaty and tired feet.
* Combats excessive perspiration and oily skin.
* Extensively used as an insect repellent.

Effects on spirit

* Uplifts the spirit.

Special precautions

* Avoid using on sensitive skin as it may cause sensitization.

Citronella is well known for its ability to deter insects. It is often used in burners and sprays. A good oil to pack in your suitcase! You can also put a drop on cotton wool and place in your drawers to deter moths.

Clary sage

Latin name: *Salvia sclarea*
Family: *Lamiaceae* (or *Labiatae*)

Principal properties and indications – keywords

* Euphoric
* Intoxicating
* Relaxing
* Tonic

Circulatory system

* Excellent for reducing the blood pressure and counteracting palpitations.

Genito-urinary system

* Recommended for childbirth since it encourages labour yet promotes relaxation.
* Tonic for the womb.
* Balances the hormones, reducing PMS.
* Relieves the pain of menstrual cramps.
* Beneficial for the menopause.

Nervous system

* Exerts a euphoric–sedative effect and indicated for overactive and panicky states of mind.
* Induces a sense of well-being and optimism and creates a padding between you and the outside world.

* Suitable for all stress-related disorders and general debility whether physical, mental, nervous or sexual.
  * Of assistance for those endeavouring to withdraw from drugs.

Skin
  * Useful for soothing and cooling inflamed skin.
  * Helps to balance oily skin, dandruff and stimulates hair growth.
  * Prevents wrinkles from occurring.

Effects on spirit
  * Valuable for instilling inner tranquillity; it uplifts the spirit.

Special precautions
  * Large doses should not be taken together with alcohol which may induce a narcotic effect.
  * Some say avoid during pregnancy, although there is no research to support or reject this.

Clary sage is the ultimate euphoric. If your mind is overactive then clary sage will banish unwanted thoughts and induce a sense of calm.

Cypress

Latin name: *Cupressus sempervirens*
Family: *Cupressaceae*

Principal properties and indications – keywords
  * Astringent   * Warming
  * Fluid-reducing   * Tonic

Circulatory system
  * Renowned for reducing varicose veins and haemorrhoids.

Genito-urinary system
  * Helpful for fluid retention.
  * Recommended for PMS and the menopause (ideal for hot flushes).
  * Regulates the menstrual cycle.

Nervous system

   * A comforting oil indicated for bereavement.
   * Relieves anger, irritability and all stress-related conditions.
   * Restores calm, balance and serenity.

Skin

   * Excellent for oily skin and for reducing excessive
     perspiration.
   * Combats cellulite.

Effects on spirit

   * Helpful for coping with change and for finding your soul
     pathway.

Special precautions

   * None.

Cypress is the oil of change – use it when moving house, changing jobs, cutting old ties or for bereavement. Blend two drops cypress and one drop lemon in 10 ml carrier oil to prevent and alleviate varicose veins.

Eucalyptus

Latin name: *Eucalyptus globulus*
Family: *Myrtaceae*

Principal properties and indications – keywords

   * Antiseptic   * Pain-relieving
   * Expectorant   * Stimulating

Circulatory system

   * Useful for poor circulation.

Genito-urinary system

   * Excellent for all urinary infections, cystitis, thrush.
   * Reduces fluid retention.

Muscular/joints

   * Excellent for all aches and pains, arthritis and rheumatism
     due to its pain-relieving properties.

Nervous system
* Combats mental exhaustion and aids concentration.
* Encourages positivity.

Respiratory system
* Very useful as an inhalant and chest rub for all respiratory disorders.
* Decongests the head and chest and helps to expel mucus.
* Enhances breathing function.
* Useful for asthma, bronchitis, coughs, colds, flu, sinusitis and throat infections.
* Reduces fever, prevents the spread of infection and boosts the immune system.

Skin
* Useful for infectious skin diseases such as chickenpox and measles.
* Recommended for herpes, cuts and burns.
* Excellent insect repellent.

Effects on spirit
* Revives the spirit and clears past traumas.

Special precautions
* A powerful oil not to be massaged into babies and very young children.
* Store away from homoeopathic medicines.

An invaluable oil for coughs and colds. Burn eucalyptus in your home to prevent the spread of infection.

Fennel (Sweet)

Latin name: *Foeniculum vulgare*
Family: *Umbelliferae* (or *Apiaceae*)

Principal properties and indications – keywords
* Detoxifying
* Digestive
* Eliminative
* Energizing
* Fluid-reducing
* Warming

Circulatory system
* Excellent as a lymphatic decongestant.

Digestive system
* Marvellous for cleansing the digestive system (and all other systems too).
* Relieves constipation, flatulence and nausea.
* A helpful aid for slimming, curbing the appetite yet increasing energy levels.

Genito-urinary system
* Excellent for nursing mothers as it increases the flow of breast milk.
* Highly effective for the menopause since it encourages the body to produce its own oestrogen.
* Regulates the menstrual cycle.
* Eases fluid retention.

Nervous system
* Encourages the ability to see a situation clearly.
* Induces courage, strength and hope in the face of seemingly impossible hurdles.
* Recommended for addictions.

Skin
* Indicated for toxic, dull, congested skin.
* Recommended for cellulite.

Effects on spirit
* Helpful for protection against psychic attack.

Special precautions
* Do not use bitter fennel.
* Do not use excessively on young children or epileptics.
* Avoid during pregnancy.

Fennel is a valuable asset when dieting as it helps to curb the appetite yet increases your energy levels. It is really detoxifying too.

Frankincense

Latin name: *Boswellia carteri*
Family: *Burseraceae*

Principal properties and indications – keywords

* Comforting
* Decongestive
* Expectorant
* Elevating
* Healing
* Rejuvenating

Genito-urinary system

* Combats cystitis.
* Useful for all vaginal discharges.
* Beneficial during the menopause.

Nervous system

* Elevating yet soothing effect on the emotions.
* Allows past traumas and anxieties to fade away.
* Instils peace and calm and is an excellent aid for meditation.
* Useful for those who fear change.
* Alleviates stress-related conditions.

Respiratory system

* Ideal for asthma and other respiratory disorders. It has both physical and emotional benefits.
* Encourages the breathing to slow down and deepen.

Skin

* Excellent remedy for all types of skin.
* Rejuvenates and revitalizes mature skin and wrinkles and helps to prevent ageing.
* Reduces scars and stretch marks.

Effects on spirit

* Valuable for achieving heightened states of spiritual awareness and bringing one closer to the Divine.

Special precautions

* None.

An excellent aid for meditation as it induces a heightened spiritual awareness. Frankincense also allows us to release, let go of the past and move on.

Geranium

Latin name: *Pelargonium graveolens*
Family: *Geraniaceae*

Principal properties and indications – keywords

* Antidepressant
* Balancing
* Fluid-reducing
* Healing
* Uplifting

Circulatory system

* Helpful for varicose veins and haemorrhoids.
* Stimulates the lymphatic system.

Genito-urinary system

* Excellent for the menopause and PMS.
* Balances the hormones and combats hot flushes.
* Reduces fluid retention.
* Helpful for cystitis.

Nervous system

* Wonderfully balancing for the nerves.
* Dispels anxiety, depression and nervous tension.
* Helps infertility problems.

Skin

* Very balancing for all types of skin – inflamed, oily, dry, combination and mature.
* Recommended for eczema, dermatitis, burns, infectious skin diseases and cellulite.
* Excellent for head lice and as an insect repellent.

Effects on spirit

* Valuable for uplifting the spirit.

Special precautions

* None.

Put a few drops on a tissue, take a few deep breaths and put it in your pocket so that you can continue to inhale the aroma throughout the day.

Ginger

Latin name: *Zingiber officinale*
Family: *Zingerberaceae*

Principal properties and indications – keywords

* Digestive
* Fiery
* Pain-relieving
* Stimulant
* Warming

Circulatory system

* Highly effective for stimulating poor circulation.

Digestive system

* Excellent for all digestive problems especially nausea (travel, chemotherapy, early morning sickness).
* Useful for diarrhoea, constipation, hangover, indigestion, flatulence, abdominal distension, loss of appetite and stomach cramps.

Muscles/joints

* Indicated for all muscular aches and pains.
* Alleviates arthritis, cramps, rheumatism, sprains and strains. Ginger works particularly well when these conditions are aggravated by damp.

Nervous system

* A warming, uplifting oil for counteracting coldness and indifference, apathy, lethargy and nervous exhaustion.
* Useful for weak-minded individuals.
* Aids concentration and memory and boosts confidence.

Respiratory system

* Excellent for coughs and colds.
* Recommended for catarrh, bronchitis, sinusitis and sore throats.

Effects on spirit
* A grounding oil which brings balance and increases our inner strength and will.

Special precautions
* Use in low dilutions if the skin is hypersensitive. At normal dosage no irritation will occur.

Ginger is well known for its warming effects and treatment of digestive problems. Use a couple of drops on a tissue or handkerchief to combat travel sickness.

Grapefruit

Latin name: *Citrus paradisi*
Family: *Rutaceae*

Principal properties and indications – keywords
* Antidepressant
* Refreshing
* Detoxifying
* Uplifting

Circulatory system
* Useful for unclogging the lymphatic system.

Digestive system
* An excellent aid to digestion and for detox diets.
* Useful for obesity, liver and gall bladder problems.
* Recommended for those who comfort eat.

Muscles/joints
* Valuable for arthritis, gout, rheumatism.
* Useful before and after exercise for preventing stiffness in the muscles and joints.

Nervous system
* Uplifts the mind, helping to lift depression and inducing euphoria.
* Helpful for dispelling bitterness and resentment.
* Beneficial for nervous exhaustion and stress relief.
* Increases self-esteem.

Respiratory system
   * Alleviates coughs, colds, flu and glandular fever.

Skin
   * Useful for oily and congested skin, acne and cellulite.

Effects on spirit
   * Uplifts the spirit.

Special precautions
   * None.

Jasmine

Latin name: *Jasminum officinale*
Family: *Oleaceae*

Principal properties and indications – keywords
   * Antidepressant   * Healing
   * Aphrodisiac   * Uplifting
   * Euphoric

Genito-urinary system
   * Highly recommended for childbirth as it helps to relieve
     pain, promote the birth and expel the placenta.
   * Useful after childbirth since it stimulates milk production
     and prevents postnatal depression.
   * A renowned aphrodisiac, jasmine can alleviate frigidity,
     impotence and premature ejaculation.
   * Increases the sperm count.
   * Excellent for painful menstruation, PMS and the menopause.

Nervous system
   * A wonderful oil for problems of the nervous system,
     releasing anxiety, lifting sadness and depression and
     inducing optimism, confidence and euphoria.

Skin
   * Excellent for all types of skin, jasmine increases the
     elasticity of the skin and reduces stretch marks and scars.

Effects on spirit
* Liberates the spirit.

Special precautions
* Do not take internally (it is an absolute).

Jasmine makes one feel optimistic and confident. Jasmine also releases inhibitions and is a powerful aphrodisiac!

Juniper berry

Latin name: *Juniperus communis*
Family: *Cupressaceae*

Principal properties and indications – keywords
* Antiseptic
* Cleansing
* Detoxifying
* Fluid-reducing
* Purifying
* Tonic

Circulatory system
* Renowned as a wonderful detoxifier.
* Beneficial for arteriosclerosis.
* Decongests the lymphatic system.

Digestive system
* Stimulates the elimination of toxins and therefore useful for obesity, constipation and stomach upsets after too much rich food and alcohol.

Genito-urinary system
* Excellent for relieving fluid retention.
* One of the best oils for urinary infections such as cystitis.
* A remedy for scanty, irregular and painful menstruation.

Muscles/joints
* Alleviates arthritis, gout and rheumatic disorders, stimulating the elimination of uric acid and other toxins and relieving pain and stiffness.

Nervous system
* Clears waste from the mind just as it does from the body.

Skin

* Recommended for all skin conditions due to an accumulation of toxins.
* Invaluable for cellulite, acne, blocked pores and oily skin.
* Helpful for dermatitis, eczema and psoriasis.

Effects on spirit

* A classic remedy for purifying and cleansing the spirit and for those who are unable to move on.
* Juniper helps to clear away the residues of unwanted past traumas.

Special precautions

* Avoid during pregnancy.
* Do not use excessively where there is inflammation of the kidneys.

Juniper clears toxins from the body, mind and spirit. Use in the bath after over-indulging and whenever you feel emotionally depleted.

Lavender

Latin name: *Lavandula angustifolia/officinalis/vera*
Family: *Lamiaceae* (or *Labiatae*)

Principal properties and indications – keywords

* Antidepressant
* Antiseptic
* Balancing
* Calming
* Healing

Circulatory system

* Excellent for high blood pressure, palpitations and all other cardiac disorders exacerbated by stress.

Digestive system

* Good for all digestive disorders, especially in children, such as colic and diarrhoea.
* Useful for difficult and painful digestion, flatulence, indigestion, nausea and vomiting.

Genito-urinary system
* Helpful for cystitis, discharges and fluid retention.
* During childbirth lavender speeds up the delivery, calms the mother and purifies the air.
* Relieves PMS, menstrual pain and the menopause.

Muscles/joints
* Reduces muscular aches and pains since lavender provides pain relief, relieves spasm and reduces inflammation.
* Recommended for arthritis, rheumatism, cramps, sprains and strains.

Nervous system
* Harmonizes the nervous system.
* Relieves emotional stress and anxiety.
* Combats depression.
* Excellent remedy for migraines, headaches and insomnia.

Respiratory system
* As an immuno-booster lavender is recommended for protection against all infections.
* Useful for viruses, colds, coughs, flu, bronchitis, asthma and throat infections.

Skin
* Useful for all skin care due to its powers of rejuvenation, antiseptic, antifungal, pain-relieving, healing and balancing properties.
* Helps to heal bruises, burns, sunburn, acne, boils, eczema, fungal infections (e.g. athlete's foot) and psoriasis.
* Useful for infectious skin conditions such as scabies and chickenpox.
* Heals wounds and sores.
* Treats insect bites (apply neat).

Effects on spirit
* Calms and soothes an angry spirit.
* Helps to centre those on the wrong spiritual pathway.

Special precautions
* None. Lavender is used extensively on babies and children.

Lavender is the most versatile of all essential oils and is a must-have for your first aid kit. Use it neat on cuts, burns and insect bites. Sprinkle a few drops on your pillow to combat insomnia.

Lemon
Latin name: *Citrus limonum*
Family: *Rutaceae*

Principal properties and indications – keywords
* Alkaline
* Antiseptic
* Detoxifying
* Fluid-reducing
* Purifying
* Tonic

Circulatory system
* Excellent tonic for the circulation.
* Boosts the immune system accelerating recovery time.
* Useful for high blood pressure and arteriosclerosis.
* Helpful for stopping bleeding, varicose veins and haemorrhoids.

Digestive system
* Highly effective for the digestion as it relieves hyperacidity, stomach ulcers and liver and gall bladder congestion.
* Ideal for obesity and detoxification.

Genito-urinary system
* An excellent diuretic relieving fluid retention.
* Combats kidney and bladder infections and thrush.

Muscles/joints
* Useful for arthritis, gout and rheumatism.

Nervous system
* Stimulates a tired and exhausted mind, encouraging clear thinking and aiding concentration.
* Restores confidence.

Respiratory system
* Relieves asthma, bronchitis, catarrh, colds, flu, laryngitis, throat infections and sinusitis.

Skin
* Effective for cleaning out cuts and wounds.
* Reduces broken capillaries.
* Useful for teenage problem skin.
* Recommended for cellulite.
* Beneficial for ageing skin, brown patches, greasy skin, boils, herpes and scabies.

Effects on spirit
* Restores strength, vitality and positivity to a depleted spirit.
* Spiritually cleansing.

Special precautions
* Avoid strong sunlight immediately after treatment.

To treat warts and verrucae simply dab one drop of lemon on to the affected area with a cotton wool bud or pad several times a day.

Lemongrass (West Indian)
Latin name: *Cymbopogon citratus*
Family: *Gramineae* (or *Poaceae*)

Principal properties and indications – keywords
* Astringent
* Revitalizing
* Refreshing
* Tonic

Circulatory system
* Excellent for stimulating the circulation.
* Valuable for the immune system, speeding up recovery time after debilitating illnesses such as glandular fever and ME.

Digestive system
* Stimulates the appetite and useful for colitis, flatulence and difficult digestion.

Genito-urinary system
  * Very useful after childbirth for aiding postnatal recovery and promoting the flow of breast milk.
  * Useful for fluid retention.

Muscles/joints
  * Excellent for improving muscle tone.
  * Relieves tired, achy legs and eliminates lactic acid.
  * Recommended for sports injuries, sprains and bruises.

Nervous system
  * Refreshing and revitalizing for the mind.
  * Banishes apathy and lethargy and lifts depression.

Skin
  * A tonic for the skin.
  * Helpful for open pores, excessive perspiration, acne, loose skin after dieting and cellulite.
  * Useful for infectious skin diseases such as scabies and measles.
  * Excellent for fungal infections such as athlete's foot.
  * Highly effective as an insect repellent.

Effects on spirit
  * Uplifting for the spirit, encouraging change and growth.

Special precautions
  * Do not use on babies and young children.
  * Take care with hypersensitive skin.

Use lemongrass to spur you into action! Great for that Monday morning feeling or to combat mental fatigue and nervous exhaustion at the end of a long hard day.

Lime

Latin name: *Citrus aurantifolia*
Family: *Rutaceae*

Principal properties and indications – keywords
  * Refreshing   * Uplifting
  * Revitalizing

Circulatory system
   * Excellent for improving the circulation.
   * Stimulates the lymphatic system.
   * Good immune booster.

Digestive system
   * Stimulates a poor appetite.
   * Relieves heartburn and indigestion.

Nervous system
   * Uplifting for those who are depressed or mentally run down.
   * Recommended for apathy and lethargy.

Respiratory system
   * A most pleasant gargle for sore throats.
   * Useful for asthma, bronchitis, catarrh, colds, coughs and flu.

Skin
   * Recommended for acne, boils, chilblains, cellulite, cuts and wounds, oily skin, mouth ulcers, warts and verrucae.

Effects on spirit
   * Uplifts and enlivens the spirit.

Special precautions
   * Avoid strong sunlight immediately after treatment.

If you feel run down and in need of a tonic it's time to reach for essential oil of lime. Use in your bath to pick you up both physically and emotionally.

Mandarin

Latin name: *Citrus reticulata*
Family: *Rutaceae*

Principal properties and indications – keywords
   * Balancing
   * Joyful
   * Revitalizing
   * Uplifting
   * Tonic

Circulatory system
* Tonic for the circulation.
* Boosts the immune system.

Digestive system
* Gentle, calming tonic for the digestive system, relieving flatulence and diarrhoea.
* Useful for stimulating a poor appetite following illness.

Nervous system
* Excellent for stress-related disorders.
* Uplifting, relieving depression and anxiety.
* Engenders feelings of joy and hopefulness.

Skin
* Recommended for the prevention of stretch marks and reduction of scarring.
* Tonic for the skin.
* Helpful for oily skin and acne.

Effects on spirit
* Encourages feelings of spiritual happiness.

Special precautions
* Avoid strong sunlight immediately after treatment.

Mandarin is a very gentle oil, therapeutic for young children, in pregnancy and for people who are frail or elderly.

Marjoram (Sweet)

Latin name: *Origanum marjorana*
Family: *Lamiaceae* (or *Labiatae*)

Principal properties and indications – keywords
* Calming
* Digestive
* Pain-relieving
* Sedative
* Warming

Circulatory system
* Excellent oil for improving the circulation and relieving chilblains.
* Regulates the heart and reduces high blood pressure.

Digestive system
* Recommended for relieving constipation, diarrhoea, flatulence, indigestion, stomach cramps and ulcers.

Genito-urinary system
* Useful for alleviating painful and irregular menstruation.
* Helps to quell excessive sexual impulses.

Muscles/joints
* Very effective for aches and pains, arthritis, rheumatism, sprains and strains.
* Alleviates pain, coldness and stiffness.

Nervous system
* Exerts a warming and comforting effect on the emotions easing grief, sadness and depression.
* Recommended for all states of anxiety.
* Useful for those individuals who are unable to sit still.

Respiratory system
* Helpful for colds and flu as an inhalation or chest rub.
* Relieves catarrh and sinusitis.
* Encourages deeper breathing.

Effects on spirit
* Excellent for fearful individuals with much agitation and who can find no peace and are constantly searching for the meaning of life.

Special precautions
* Avoid during pregnancy (although adverse effects are extremely unlikely).

This comforting sedative oil is recommended for all states of anxiety. It is particularly useful for the recently bereaved and broken hearted as it instils peace and creates a 'padding' between you and the outside world.

Myrrh

Latin name: *Commiphora myrrha*
Family: *Burseraceae*

Principal properties and indications – keywords

* Antiseptic
* Anticatarrhal
* Healing
* Rejuvenating

Digestive system

* Relieves flatulence, indigestion, diarrhoea, irritable bowel syndrome and haemorrhoids.

Genito-urinary system

* A cleanser of the womb, effective for thrush and vaginal discharges of all descriptions.
* Recommended for scanty and painful menstruation.

Nervous system

* Helpful for weak-minded individuals who are apathetic, lethargic and difficult to spur into action.
* Instils calmness and tranquillity.
* Combats worry and over-thinking.

Respiratory system

* Highly effective for respiratory problems such as asthma, bronchitis, catarrh and coughs.
* Dries up mucus.
* Helpful as a gargle for sore throats and loss of voice.

Skin

* Rejuvenates mature and wrinkled skin.
* Heals cracked, chapped and weepy skin.
* Combats fungal infections such as athlete's foot.

Effects on spirit

* Helpful for those who see life as a series of negative obstacles.

Special precautions
* Avoid during pregnancy (although there is no research to support or reject this).

To banish mouth ulcers and also gum infections such as gingivitis try gargling with two drops of myrrh in half a glass of water.

Neroli (Orange blossom)

Latin name: *Citrus aurantium* var. *amara*
Family: *Rutaceae*

Principal properties and indications – keywords
* Antidepressant
* Aphrodisiac
* Sedative
* Stress-relieving

Circulatory system
* Excellent for high blood pressure, palpitations, false angina and nervous heart conditions.

Digestive system
* Highly effective for colitis, chronic diarrhoea and nervous indigestion.

Genito-urinary system
* Useful for the menopause and PMS.

Nervous system
* Valuable for all nervous problems, chronic and short-term anxiety and panic attacks.
* Lifts depression and instils a feeling of euphoria.
* Relieves insomnia.
* Its aphrodisiacal properties make it ideal for sexual problems such as impotence and frigidity caused by tension and apprehension.

Skin
* Wonderful oil for all types of skin.
* Encourages the regeneration of skin cells and works wonders for mature skins.

* Recommended for preventing stretch marks and reducing scars.
* Ideal for sensitive skins.

Effects on spirit
* Puts us in touch with our higher selves.

Special precautions
* None.

Neroli is one of the most beautiful and effective oils for treating stress. It is an expensive oil but worth the investment. Neroli is also a renowned aphrodisiac – why not try sprinkling a few drops on your bed linen?

Patchouli

Latin name: *Pogostemon patchouli/cablin*
Family: *Lamiaceae* (or *Labiatae*)

Principal properties and indications – keywords
* Antidepressant
* Healing
* Hypnotizing
* Rejuvenating
* Soothing

Digestive system
* Curbs the appetite and is useful for those who are trying to lose weight.
* Useful for relieving constipation, diarrhoea and irritable bowel syndrome.
* Tones the colon and relieves bloatedness.

Nervous system
* Popular in the 1960s possibly due to its ability to instil peace, calm and love while at the same time helping to clarify problems.
* Beneficial for all stress-related problems and sexual problems.
* Lifts depression.

Skin

* Encourages the regeneration of skin cells and is recommended for mature skin and scar tissue.
* Heals chapped and cracked skin and soothes and cools down skin redness.
* Tones up loose skin after dieting.
* Useful for fungal infections such as athlete's foot and allergies such as eczema.

Effects on spirit

* Exerts a grounding effect on those who feel detached from their bodies.

Special precautions

* None.

The musky aroma of patchouli acts as a powerful aphrodisiac. To stimulate sexual desire sprinkle a few drops in an oil burner and allow the sensual aroma to diffuse into the atmosphere.

Peppermint

Latin name: *Mentha piperita*
Family: *Lamiaceae* (or *Labiatae*)

Principal properties and indications – keywords

* Cooling
* Digestive
* Pain relieving
* Stimulating
* Tonic

Digestive system

* Recommended for all digestive problems, alleviating nausea and travel sickness.
* Useful for diarrhoea, constipation, indigestion and flatulence.
* Excellent for pain relief.

Muscles/joints

* Favourable for general pain relief relieving muscular aches, arthritis, neuralgia and rheumatism. One drop in a glass of water may be taken instead of aspirin.

* Exerts a cooling and anaesthetic action when used as a compress on headaches and migraine.

Nervous system
* Stimulates the mind, eliminating mental fatigue and encouraging concentration.
* Recommended in times of crisis as peppermint strengthens yet numbs the nerves.

Skin
* Cools down sunburn and relieves itching and inflammation.
* Helpful for toxic, congested skin and acne.
* Useful for infectious skin conditions such as ringworm and scabies.

Effects on spirit
* Helps to wake up, revive and stimulate the spirit into action.

Special precautions
* Store away from homoeopathic medications and do not use in conjunction with homoeopathic treatment.
* Avoid using when breastfeeding as it halts lactation.
* Take care with sensitive skins (although irritation is rare).
* Do not use on babies and young children.

Peppermint is a great pain reliever and is very cooling. Try a peppermint compress to relieve muscular aches and joint pains. A cold compress of peppermint and lavender placed on the forehead or the back of the neck is a good way to reduce a fever.

Rose

Latin names: *Rosa damascena (Damask rose/Bulgarian rose/ Turkish rose) Rosa centifolia (Cabbage/Moroccan rose)*

Family: *Rosaceae*

Principal properties and indications – keywords
* Antidepressant
* Aphrodisiac
* Balancing
* Rejuvenating
* Uplifting

Circulatory system

* Purifying for the blood and is an excellent tonic for the heart.
* Reduces palpitations.

Genito-urinary system

* This 'queen' of oils has a remarkable effect on disorders of the female reproductive system.
* Cleanses, regulates and tones the womb.
* Recommended for PMS and the menopause.
* Renowned as an aphrodisiac and recommended for impotence and frigidity.
* Aids conception and increases the production of semen.

Nervous system

* The exquisite, luxurious aroma has a profound effect on the emotions, alleviating grief, anger, jealousy, resentment, stress and tension.
* Makes a woman feel feminine and positive.
* Recommended for all states of depression.
* Dissolves psychological pain.

Skin

* Excellent for all types of skin, especially dry, mature or sensitive.
* Calms down inflammation and reduces broken thread veins.

Effects on spirit

* Particularly beneficial for a closed heart, encouraging love and compassion.
* Releases past traumas.

Special precautions

* Can be used safely with children.

Rose instils harmony and positivity and is well worth the investment. Instead of sending a bunch of roses send a bottle of rose oil!

Rosemary

Latin name: *Rosmarinus officinalis*
Family: *Lamiaceae* (or *Labiatae*)

Principal properties and indications – keywords

* Diuretic
* Pain relieving
* Restorative
* Stimulating

Circulatory system

* Excellent for poor circulation and congestion in the lymphatic system.
* Tonic for the heart, normalizing blood cholesterol levels and arteriosclerosis.

Digestive system

* Valuable for many digestive complaints, particularly if detoxification is required.
* Useful for constipation, flatulence, liver congestion, food poisoning and obesity.

Genito-urinary system

* Recommended for combating fluid retention, discharges, cystitis and painful or scanty menstruation.

Muscles/joints

* Highly recommended for pain relief in muscles and joints, easing arthritis, rheumatism and stiff, overworked muscles.
* Useful for poor muscle tone.

Nervous system

* Activates and enlivens the brain, clearing the head and reducing mental fatigue.
* Useful for memory loss and for reviving the senses of smell, speech and hearing.

Respiratory system

* Beneficial for asthma, bronchitis, catarrh, colds, flu and whooping cough.

Skin

* Use for toxic, congested skin and infectious conditions such as scabies.
* Reduces cellulite.
* A traditional ingredient of hair care preparations encouraging hair growth, relieving dandruff and combating head lice.

Effects on spirit

* Excellent for 'loss' of spirit.

Special precautions

* Do not use extensively in the first stages of pregnancy (although side-effects are highly unlikely).
* Do not use extensively on epileptics.

Rosemary is the great restorer! It awakens the brain, improves the memory and greatly improves energy levels. A marvellous oil to use in your bath/shower first thing in the morning.

Sandalwood

Latin name: *Santalum album*
Family: *Santalaceae*

Principal properties and indications – keywords

* Aphrodisiac	* Soothing
* Healing	* Uplifting

Circulatory system

* Tonic for the heart, exerting a sedative yet regulatory effect.

Genito-urinary system

* Highly effective at alleviating cystitis and vaginal infections of all kinds.
* Reduces fluid retention.

Nervous system

* Renowned for its balancing effect on the nervous system, gently soothing away anxiety and tension.

* Combats insomnia.
* Recommended as an aphrodisiac and therefore ideal for impotence and frigidity.

Respiratory system
* Beneficial for chest infections, coughs, bronchitis and sore throats.

Skin
* Used extensively for all skin complaints, especially dry, cracked and dehydrated skin.
* Recommended as an aftershave when blended with a carrier oil.

Effects on spirit
* Brings peace and tranquillity to the troubled soul.
* Recommended for meditation.

Special precautions
* None.

Sandalwood is renowned for its ability to soothe away stress and anxiety. Use it in the bath to gently take away your worries and fears. Sandalwood is one of my favourites for meditation as it creates a sense of profound peace.

Tea tree

Latin name: *Melaleuca alternifolia*
Family: *Myrtaceae*

Principal properties and indications – keywords
* Antifungal
* Antiseptic
* First aid
* Stimulating

Circulatory system
* Tonic for the heart stimulating the circulation and reducing varicose veins.
* Highly recommended as an immuno-booster and therefore may help to combat repeated infections, glandular fever and postviral syndrome, myalgia encephalomyelitis (ME).

Genito-urinary system
* Excellent for cystitis, itching, thrush and vaginal discharges and infections.

Nervous system
* After an emotional crisis tea tree may be used to ease the shock.

Respiratory system
* Beneficial for asthma, bronchitis, catarrh, colds, flu, sinusitis, and whooping cough.
* Ideal as a gargle for throat infections.

Skin
* Valuable for acne, athlete's foot, boils, burns, cuts, herpes, itching, spots and sweaty or smelly feet.
* May be applied neat to warts and verrucae.
* Recommended for problems with toenails.
* Useful for mouth ulcers and cold sores.

Effects on spirit
* Helps to clear old traumas.

Special precautions
* None. Tea tree is often used neat for first aid purposes.

Tea tree is the 'first aid kit' in a bottle. Always take a bottle when travelling for dabbing on cuts and insect bites. Great for warts and verrucae too – apply one drop to the affected area two to three times daily until it disappears.

Thyme

Latin name: *Thymus vulgaris*
Family: *Lamiaceae* (or *Labiatae*)

Principal properties and indications – keywords
* Antiseptic   * Stimulant
* Energizing

Circulatory system
* Stimulates the circulation and it may be used to raise blood pressure.
* An excellent booster of the immune system.
* Benefits chronic fatigue.
* Useful for convalescence.

Digestive system
* Cleanses the digestive system.
* Eases abdominal distension, candida and flatulence.
* Restores the appetite.

Genito-urinary system
* Useful for fluid retention, urinary infections and vaginal discharges.

Muscles/joints
* Recommended for sports injuries.
* Eases gout, rheumatism and arthritis.

Nervous system
* Reviving and energizing oil which stimulates the mind and improves the memory and powers of concentration.
* Beneficial for nervous depression.

Respiratory system
* Helpful for asthma, bronchitis, catarrh, colds, coughs, sinusitis.
* Excellent (as a gargle) for throat, mouth and gum infections.

Skin
* Useful for treating head lice and scabies.
* Helpful for skin infection.

Effects on spirit
* Revives a tired spirit and helps to release blockages caused by past traumas.

Special precautions
* Avoid taking during pregnancy.
* Take care with sensitive skin.
* Do not use excessively in cases of high blood pressure.
* Do not use on babies and young children.

If you suffer with low blood pressure thyme is a must-have – sprinkle a couple of drops on to a tissue and inhale several times a day.

Vetivert

Latin name: *Andropogon muricatus/Vetiveria zizaniodes*
Family: *Gramineae* (or *Poaceae*)

Principal properties and indications – keywords
* Calming
* Tranquillizing
* Protective

Circulatory system
* Stimulates the circulation.
* Tonic for the immune system.

Digestive system
* Useful for a poor appetite.
* Helpful for IBS.

Genito-urinary system
* Useful for PMS.
* Recommended during the menopause.

Muscles/joints
* Recommended as a muscle relaxant.
* Alleviates arthritis, rheumatism, cramps, sprains and strains.

Nervous system
* This 'oil of tranquillity' has a profoundly sedative effect and may be useful for those who are trying to stop taking tranquillizers or other addictive substances.
* Useful for deep psychological problems and hypochondriacs.
* Helpful for insomnia.

Effects on spirit
* Excellent for those who feel out of balance or ungrounded.
* Useful as a protective shield where individuals are oversensitive.

Special precautions
* None.

The earthy aroma of vetivert, so reminiscent of roots, is perfect for when you feel ungrounded and have that 'out of the body' feeling. Put a drop on a tissue and inhale deeply to bring yourself back to earth.

Ylang ylang
Latin name: *Cananga odorata* var. *genuina*
Family: *Annonaceae*

Principal properties and indications – keywords
* Antidepressant
* Aphrodisiac
* Euphoric
* Soothing

Circulatory system
* Reduces high blood pressure and has a regulatory effect on the heart.
* Helpful for palpitations, rapid heartbeat (tachycardia) and rapid breathing (hyperpnoea).

Nervous system
* Deeply relaxing, releasing anxiety, tension, anger and fear.
* Uplifts depression and creates a sense of euphoria.
* Restores confidence.
* Relieves insomnia and thoughts that go round and round in the mind.
* Powerful aphrodisiac.
* Recommended for epilepsy.

Skin
* Used extensively for all skin care – both oily and dry skins benefit.
* Promotes hair growth.

Effects on spirit
    * Brings peace to the troubled spirit.

Special precautions
    * None.

Ylang ylang is extremely sensuous and is a powerful aphrodisiac. Light a couple of candles in your bedroom, wait until the wax has slightly melted and then put one or two drops into the melted wax, avoiding the wick.

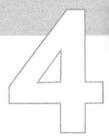

aromamassage

Massage is a highly therapeutic tool in its own right, so when massage is used in combination with the healing qualities of essential oils, it is a powerful tool for restoring physical, emotional and spiritual levels. During an aromamassage, emotions may be released alongside the accumulated knots and nodules. The tissues and the nervous system are able to 'remember' both physical and emotional trauma.

One of the most rewarding things you can do is to give a healing aromamassage to the back, legs, feet, abdomen or face of family members and friends. Why not swap an aromamassage once a week with a friend and notice the improvement in your health and well being?

Setting the scene

To derive maximum benefit from the treatment it is important to pay attention to the environment in which the aromamassage is to be performed. Both the giver and the receiver should feel immediately relaxed. An aromamassage should never be hurried.

Solitude and quiet

These are vital. Ensure that you choose a time when you will not be disturbed. Take the telephone off the hook. You may decide to choose some soothing background music although this is a matter of personal preference; some will prefer silence.

Cleanliness

This is essential. Always wash your hands before the treatment, as any stickiness will be instantly obvious to the receiver. Make sure that your fingernails are short – trim them as far down as possible. Do not wear any jewellery on your hands. Rings, bracelets and watches can all scratch the receiver.

Warmth

The room should be draught-free and warm yet well ventilated. The room in which you give the aromamassage should be heated prior to treatment and, as the receiver's body temperature will drop, ensure that spare towels are at your disposal. Warm your hands if they feel cold.

Keep all areas of the receiver's body covered, other than the part on which you are working. The receiver should be kept warm at all times.

Lighting

Soft and subdued lighting will create the ideal atmosphere. Bright lights falling on the receiver's face will hardly induce relaxation and will cause tension around his or her eyes. Candlelight provides the perfect setting, or you may wish to use a tinted bulb.

Colour

The most therapeutic colours to have in the room are pastel shades – pale pink, blue, green or peach decor and towels are perfect for the occasion. Strong colours such as red will tend to create unwanted emotions like anger and restlessness.

Clothes

Wear comfortable and loose-fitting clothes as you need to move around easily and the room in which you will be working will be warm. White is the best colour to wear when giving an aromamassage since it will reflect any negativity which is released from the individual being treated.

Wear flat shoes or, even better, go barefoot. The receiver should undress down to whatever level he or she feels comfortable with. Suggest undressing down to the underwear. Point out that areas which are not being worked on will be covered up as this will create a sense of security and trust.

Finishing touches

Fresh flowers add a pleasant aroma to the atmosphere, or you can burn incense or essential oils prior to the treatment.

Equipment

Aromamassage surface

Work on the floor using a firm yet well-padded surface. Place a large, thick piece of foam, two or three blankets or a thick duvet on the floor. Use plenty of cushions or pillows during the treatment. When the receiver is lying on his or her back, place one pillow under the head and one under the knees to take the pressure off the back. When the receiver is lying on his or her front, place a pillow under the feet, one under the head and shoulders and one under the abdomen, if desired.

Ensure that you have something to kneel on to avoid sore knees. If you are unfortunate enough to suffer from back or knee problems it may be a good idea to invest in a portable couch. It is far less tiring and makes the receiver's body readily accessible. You could try improvising by using a kitchen table if the height is comfortable for you.

Do not use a bed as most are far too soft and wide for massage purposes and any pressure applied is absorbed by the mattress. Also a bed will not be the right height for your back.

Your attitude and state of mind

Posture

Whether you are working on the floor or at a table, keep your back relaxed yet straight throughout the aromamassage. When standing bend your knees slightly and tuck your bottom in so that your back can work from a secure base (i.e. the pelvis). Allow your thighs to do most of the work – not your back. Remember that it should be as relaxing to give a massage as it is to receive one.

Attunement

Your state of mind when giving an aromamassage is vital. The quality and success of a treatment depends upon having a calm state of mind. Your complete attention must be devoted to the receiver. If you are worrying about your own problems and your mind is drifting, this will be communicated immediately. Make sure that you are aware of the receiver's breathing and that you are sensitive to his or her reactions. Observe facial expressions and be aware of any tensing up in the muscles.

Spend time consciously relaxing yourself prior to the treatment and, most importantly, be guided by your own intuition. Take a few deep breaths before the aromamassage allowing all tension and anxiety to flow out of your body. Breathe in peace and breathe out love. Tune in to the person you are massaging. It may help to work with your eyes closed.

Contraindications

As a general rule, most essential oils are safe provided they are used properly and sensibly. However, please observe the following points at all times.

* Do not apply essential oils to the skin undiluted (except for lavender and tea tree for first-aid purposes) as they are far too concentrated and can result in inflammation and allergic reaction.
* Keep oils away from the eyes.
* Keep oils out of reach of children.
* Ensure that the dosage is accurate as too much essential oil can be harmful.
* Purchase only pure essential oils.
* Take care with particularly sensitive skins – it is possible to do a patch test if you are anxious.
* Do not massage where there is a high fever. The body has already raised itself to a high temperature to fight off the infection and does not need the burden of even more toxins to deal with. However, essential oils may be applied on compresses in order to reduce temperature.
* Do not massage the abdomen heavily during pregnancy, especially for the first three months where risk of miscarriage is at its highest. Beware of certain oils throughout pregnancy. Check that there are no special precautions for any of your chosen oils.
* Beware of infectious skin conditions (e.g. scabies), although aromatherapy baths and blended creams are recommended.
* Use only light pressure over severe varicose veins.
* Beware of recent scar tissue, open wounds and areas of inflammation.
* Beware of unexplained lumps and bumps – always have them investigated by a doctor.
* Avoid areas of inflammation (e.g. bursitis – 'housemaid's knee').
* Avoid exposure to strong sunshine or sunbeds immediately after an aromatherapy massage.

* Wait a couple of hours after a sauna as the pores are open and the body is still eliminating.

The treatment

Space does not permit me to describe a complete aromatherapy treatment. However, the following sequence will enable you to perform a few simple movements so that you can treat your family and friends.

The back

Aromamassage of the back may be used to aid relaxation and release the tense and knotted muscles brought about by factors such as stress, poor posture and a sedentary lifestyle. It can also relieve constipation and menstrual and respiratory problems.

The receiver should lie on his or her front with one pillow under the feet, one under the head, and one under the abdomen if desired.

1 Start with both hands relaxed at the base of the receiver's back, one hand either side of the spine. Stroke both hands up the back using your bodyweight to apply pressure, spread your hands across the shoulders and then allow them to glide back gently. Repeat this movement as often as you like, to promote deep relaxation.

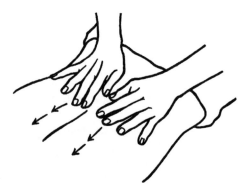

Stroke the back.

2 Starting at the base of the spine, make small, circular movements with your thumbs until you reach the neck (friction movements). Do not press directly on to the spine itself. Now perform these circular movements around each shoulder blade to loosen the knots and nodules.

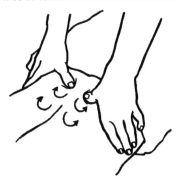

Friction up the back from the base of the spine to the neck.

3 Repeat step 1.

4 Step 4 is performed along the sides of the body and aims to drain away the toxins, both physical and emotional. Place both hands at the base of the spine on the side opposite you. Work up one side of the back pushing the toxins down towards the couch or the floor and gently flick them away. Repeat on the other side.

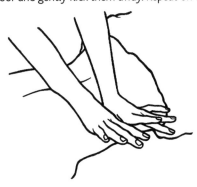

Drain the toxins.

5 To release tension from the shoulders work across the top of them, alternately picking up and gently squeezing the tense muscles. This movement is called 'wringing' and if you are good at making bread this movement will come easily to you.

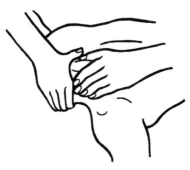

Wring across the tops of the shoulders.

6 To finish the back repeat the stroking movements as in step 1.

The legs

Aromamassage of the legs can be used to improve the circulation of the blood and lymph (to cleanse away toxins), relieve cramp and combat fluid retention and it helps alleviate and prevent varicose veins.

1 Position yourself at the feet of the receiver. Beginning at the ankle stroke up towards the thigh with one hand in front of the other. Use no pressure on the way down.

2 To reduce tension from the muscles and to encourage the release of toxins accumulated in the deeper tissues, knead the muscular areas on the calf and thigh. Place both hands flat down and squeeze and pick up the muscles with alternate hands.

3 Repeat step 1.

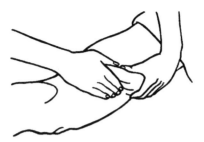

Wring the thigh and calf muscles.

The feet

Regular aromamassage of the feet can dramatically improve the circulation, relieve aches and pains and maintain flexibility and suppleness. It is also wonderfully relaxing and soothing.

1 Stroke the foot firmly covering the top, sides and sole, working from the ends of the toes towards the ankle. Slide around the ankle bones and glide back to your starting position.
2 Support the foot with one hand and use the knuckles of the other hand (lightly clenched fist) to circle firmly over the entire sole of the foot.
3 Repeat step 1 as many times as you like.

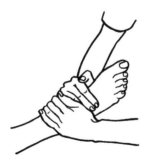

Stroke the foot firmly.

The abdomen

Aromamassage of the abdomen is excellent for relieving digestive problems such as bloating and constipation and for menstrual problems such as PMT.

Aromamassage of the abdomen is easy to perform. Position yourself on the right-hand side of the receiver and massage in a clockwise direction, circling around the abdomen with one hand following the other. You are following the direction of the colon.

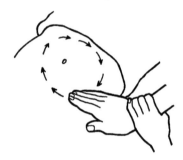

Stroke the abdomen, working in a clockwise direction.

The face

Aromamassage of the face is deeply relaxing and wonderfully uplifting. It can help to relieve skin problems, headaches, nasal problems such as sinusitis, slow down the ageing process and encourage clarity of thought.

1 Position yourself at the receiver's head and begin by stroking smoothly across the brow. Stroke outwards across the cheeks and then stroke outwards across the chin.
2 Place your thumbs at the centre of the forehead just between the eyebrows, press down and hold for two seconds. Lift your thumbs and place them slightly further out along the brow bone and repeat the pressure. Continue until you have reached the outer corners of the eyes. Work the whole forehead as far as the hairline.
3 Repeat step 1.

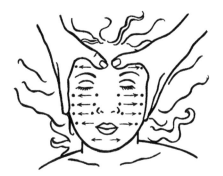

Work across the face in strips using pressure points.

4 Repeat step 2 on the cheeks and chin.
5 Spread out your fingers and thumbs and place the pads on the receiver's scalp. Circle them slowly and firmly, working gradually over the whole of the scalp area.
6 To complete your treatment stroke the hair from the roots to the tips and allow your hands to rest gently on the temples.

5

aromatherapy for common ailments: a therapeutic index

Most of the common ailments that you will ever suffer from can be treated using essential oils and they can be used in many ways, as we saw in Chapter 1.

Try to remember the following guidelines when using essential oils:

Bath – 6 drops
Shower (footbath/hand bath/sitz bath) – 6 drops
Gargles/Mouthwashes – 2 drops
Steam inhalation – 3 drops
Oil burner – 6 drops
Massage – 3 drops to 10 mls

It is worth remembering that some methods may be more suited to particular conditions. For example, if you have a headache, a cooling lavender compress would bring immediate relief, whereas for sinusitis a eucalyptus inhalation would be excellent. If you were suffering from aches and pains, an aromabath or an aromamassage would be most effective.

Circulatory/immune systems

Anaemia black pepper, carrot seed, chamomile, geranium, lemon, lime, peppermint, rosemary, thyme

Arteriosclerosis black pepper, ginger, juniper, lemon, rosemary

Chilblains black pepper, ginger, lemon, marjoram

Fever black pepper, chamomile, eucalyptus, ginger, juniper, lavender, peppermint

Glandular fever cypress, lavender, lemon, tea tree, thyme

Haemorrhoids cypress, geranium, juniper, lemon, myrrh

Heart *False angina*: neroli; *Irregular heartbeat* (tachycardia): marjoram, sandalwood, ylang ylang; *Tonic*: benzoin, lavender, marjoram, neroli, rose, sandalwood

High blood pressure chamomile, clary sage, lavender, lemon, marjoram, neroli, ylang ylang

High cholesterol ginger, juniper, lemon, rosemary, thyme

Immune system booster carrot seed, chamomile, lavender, lemon, lemongrass, lime, mandarin, tea tree, thyme, vetivert

Low blood pressure rosemary, thyme

Lymphatic congestion carrot seed, cypress, fennel, grapefruit, juniper, lemon, lime, mandarin, rosemary

ME (myalgic encephalomyelitis) cypress, grapefruit, lavender, lemongrass, rosemary, tea tree, thyme

Palpitations chamomile, clary sage, lavender, neroli, rose, rosemary, ylang ylang

Poor circulation benzoin, black pepper, carrot seed, cypress, eucalyptus, ginger, lemon, lemongrass, lime, mandarin, marjoram, rosemary, thyme

Varicose veins cypress, geranium, ginger, lemon, neroli

Digestive system

Anorexia bergamot, black pepper, carrot seed, fennel, frankincense, jasmine, lavender, neroli, rose, thyme

Appetite balancer fennel, patchouli

Bulimia bergamot, clary sage, geranium, jasmine, lavender, neroli, rose

Candida chamomile, citronella, ginger, myrrh, patchouli, rosemary, tea tree, thyme

Constipation black pepper, carrot seed, fennel, ginger, marjoram, patchouli, rose, rosemary, thyme

Diabetes eucalyptus, geranium, juniper

Diarrhoea black pepper, cajeput, chamomile, cypress, eucalyptus, geranium, ginger, lavender, lemon, mandarin, myrrh, neroli (*stress induced*), patchouli, peppermint, rosemary, sandalwood

Flatulence basil, bergamot, black pepper, carrot seed, chamomile, fennel, ginger, juniper, lavender, lemon, lemongrass, mandarin, marjoram, myrrh, neroli, peppermint, rosemary, thyme

Food poisoning black pepper, fennel, grapefruit, juniper, rosemary

Hangover fennel, juniper, rosemary

Halitosis (bad breadth) bergamot, fennel, lemon, peppermint

Hiccoughs basil, fennel, mandarin

Indigestion and heartburn basil, bergamot, cajeput, chamomile, fennel, ginger, juniper, lavender, lemon, lemongrass, lime, mandarin, marjoram, neroli (*nervous*), peppermint, rosemary

IBS (irritable bowel syndrome) carrot seed, chamomile, ginger, myrrh, neroli, patchouli

Loss of appetite bergamot, black pepper, fennel, ginger, juniper, lime, peppermint, thyme

Nausea and vomiting basil, black pepper, chamomile, fennel, ginger, lavender, peppermint

Obesity black pepper, cypress, fennel, ginger, grapefruit, juniper, lemon, rosemary

Stomach pains chamomile, fennel, ginger, lavender, marjoram, peppermint, rosemary

Travel sickness ginger, mandarin, peppermint

Genito-urinary system

Childbirth clary sage, jasmine, lavender, neroli, palmarosa

Cystitis bergamot, cajeput, carrot seed, chamomile, cypress, eucalyptus, frankincense, geranium, juniper, lavender, lemon, sandalwood, tea tree

Discharges bergamot, lavender, marjoram, myrrh, rose, rosemary, sandalwood, tea tree, thyme

Excessive sexual impulses marjoram

Fluid retention benzoin, carrot seed, chamomile, cypress, eucalyptus, fennel, geranium, juniper, lavender, lemon, lemongrass, rosemary, sandalwood, thyme

Frigidity and impotence clary sage, ginger, jasmine, neroli, rose, sandalwood, ylang ylang

Infertility geranium, jasmine, rose

Insufficiency of milk in nursing mothers fennel, jasmine, lemongrass

Itching (vaginal) bergamot, chamomile, tea tree

Menopause bergamot, carrot seed, chamomile, clary sage, cypress, fennel, frankincense, geranium, jasmine, lavender, neroli, rose, sandalwood, ylang ylang

Menstruation *Heavy blood loss*: chamomile, cypress, geranium, rose, *Irregular*: chamomile, marjoram, rose, *Painful*: cajeput, chamomile, clary sage, cypress, jasmine, juniper, lavender, marjoram, myrrh, peppermint, rose, rosemary, *Scanty*:

chamomile, clary sage, fennel, juniper, lavender, marjoram, myrrh, peppermint, rose, rosemary, thyme

PMS carrot seed, chamomile, clary sage, cypress, geranium, lavender, marjoram, neroli, rose, rosemary, sandalwood, ylang ylang

Thrush bergamot, eucalyptus, frankincense, lavender, lemon, myrrh, tea tree, thyme

Urinary infections bergamot, cajeput, eucalyptus, juniper, sandalwood, tea tree, thyme

Head disorders

Catarrh basil, black pepper, cajeput, eucalyptus, frankincense, lavender, lemon, lime, myrrh, tea tree

Cold sores bergamot, chamomile, lavender, lemon, myrrh, tea tree

Earache basil, chamomile, lavender

Fainting and vertigo basil, black pepper, lavender, peppermint, rosemary

Gum infections (e.g. gingivitis) chamomile, lemon, myrrh, tea tree, thyme

Hair and scalp *Dandruff*: carrot seed, chamomile, cypress, juniper, lavender, lemon, patchouli, tea tree, thyme; *Dry*: carrot seed, geranium, lavender, rosemary, sandalwood; *Lice*: bergamot, eucalyptus, geranium, lavender, lemon, rosemary, tea tree; *Loss of hair*: chamomile, clary sage, frankincense, geranium, ginger, lavender, rosemary, *Oily*: bergamot, clary sage, cypress, frankincense, geranium, lemon, lemongrass, juniper, rosemary, thyme, *Sensitive scalp*: chamomile, lavender

Headaches and migraine basil, chamomile, lavender, marjoram, peppermint, rosemary

Loss of smell rosemary

Mouth infections and ulcers lemon, myrrh, tea tree, thyme

Neuralgia basil, black pepper, chamomile, eucalyptus, geranium, peppermint

Rhinitis and sinusitis basil, cajeput, eucalyptus, lavender, peppermint, tea tree, thyme

Toothache cajeput, chamomile, peppermint

Muscular/joint disorders

Aches and pains basil, benzoin, black pepper, cajeput, chamomile, eucalyptus, frankincense, ginger, juniper, lavender, lemon, lemongrass, lime, marjoram, peppermint, rosemary, vetivert

Arthritis basil, benzoin, black pepper, cajeput, chamomile, eucalyptus, ginger, grapefruit, juniper, lavender, lemon, marjoram, peppermint, rosemary, thyme, vetivert

Bruises black pepper, chamomile, geranium, lavender, marjoram, myrrh, peppermint, rosemary

Cramp basil, black pepper, chamomile, ginger, lavender, marjoram, rosemary, vetivert

Fibrositis benzoin, black pepper, eucalyptus, lavender, peppermint, rosemary

Gout basil, benzoin, cajeput, chamomile, grapefruit, juniper, lemon, lime, rosemary, thyme

Inflammation chamomile, lavender

Lack of muscle tone black pepper, lavender, lemongrass, rosemary

Rheumatism basil, black pepper, cajeput, chamomile, eucalyptus, frankincense, ginger, grapefruit, juniper, lavender, lemon, lime, marjoram, myrrh, peppermint, rosemary, thyme, vetivert

Sprains and strains black pepper, cajeput, chamomile, eucalyptus, ginger, lavender, lemongrass, marjoram, peppermint, rosemary, vetivert

Stiffness black pepper, chamomile, eucalyptus, frankincense, grapefruit, lavender, marjoram, rosemary

Nervous system

Alcoholism clary sage, fennel, juniper (*detoxify*), vetivert

Apathy and lethargy ginger, grapefruit, jasmine, lemongrass, lime, mandarin, myrrh, patchouli, rosemary

Change cypress (*enables acceptance*), frankincense (*enables moving on*)

Coldness benzoin, black pepper, frankincense, marjoram, rose

Comfort benzoin, black pepper, cypress, marjoram, rose

Confidence (lack of) black pepper, ginger, jasmine

Courage black pepper, fennel, ginger

Depression basil, bergamot, chamomile, clary sage, geranium, grapefruit, jasmine, lavender, lemongrass, lime, mandarin, neroli, patchouli, rose, sandalwood, thyme, ylang ylang

Exhaustion benzoin (*mental, emotional, physical*), clary sage (*nervous, physical, sexual*), citronella, eucalyptus, grapefruit, juniper (*emotional and nervous depletion*), lavender, lemon, lime, thyme

Fearful clary sage, frankincense, jasmine, lavender, neroli, sandalwood, ylang ylang

Frigidity and impotence clary sage, ginger, jasmine, neroli, patchouli, peppermint, rose, rosewood, sandalwood, ylang ylang

Grief benzoin, cypress, frankincense, mandarin, marjoram, neroli, rose

Hysteria and panic chamomile, clary sage, lavender, marjoram, neroli

Inability to concentrate basil, cajeput, lemon, peppermint, rosemary

Indecision basil, carrot seed, patchouli

Insomnia chamomile, lavender, mandarin, marjoram, neroli, rose, sandalwood, ylang ylang

Irritability chamomile, cypress, lavender, thyme

Jealousy rose

Loneliness benzoin, rose

Memory basil, black pepper, ginger, juniper, rosemary, thyme

Mental fatigue (*clears the mind*) basil, peppermint, rosemary

Mood swings chamomile, geranium, lavender

Negativity jasmine, juniper, mandarin, vetivert

Nervous tension basil, clary sage, cypress, geranium, grapefruit, lavender, mandarin, marjoram, neroli, patchouli, rose, sandalwood

Obsessions frankincense, vetivert

Over-sensitivity basil, black pepper, chamomile, cypress, geranium, lavender

Resentment grapefruit

Sadness benzoin, jasmine, rose

Sedative bergamot, chamomile, clary sage, frankincense, marjoram, sandalwood, vetivert

Shock benzoin, mandarin, neroli, peppermint, rose, ylang ylang

Respiratory system

Asthma basil, benzoin, cajeput, cypress, eucalyptus, frankincense, lavender, lemon, lime, myrrh, peppermint, rosemary, thyme

Bronchitis basil, benzoin, cajeput, cypress, eucalyptus, fennel, frankincense, ginger, lavender, lemon, lime, myrrh, peppermint, rosemary, sandalwood, tea tree, thyme

Catarrh basil, benzoin, black pepper, cajeput, eucalyptus, frankincense, ginger, lavender, lemon, myrrh, rosemary, sandalwood, tea tree

Coughs and colds benzoin, bergamot, black pepper, cajeput, eucalyptus, frankincense, ginger, grapefruit, lavender, lemon, lime, myrrh, peppermint, rosemary, sandalwood, tea tree, thyme

Emphysema eucalyptus, frankincense

Flu benzoin, bergamot, black pepper, eucalyptus, fennel, frankincense, ginger, grapefruit, lavender, lemon, lime, peppermint, rosemary, tea tree

Hoarseness and loss of voice myrrh, sandalwood

Sinusitis basil, cajeput, eucalyptus, lavender, lemon, myrtle, tea tree, thyme

Tonsillitis and throat infections benzoin, bergamot, cajeput, eucalyptus, geranium, ginger, lavender, lemon, lime, myrrh, sandalwood

Skin

Acne bergamot, carrot seed, chamomile, cypress, frankincense, grapefruit, juniper, lavender, lemon, lemongrass, lime, mandarin, patchouli, peppermint, rosemary, sandalwood, tea tree, ylang ylang

Ageing skin clary sage, frankincense, lavender, lemon, myrrh, neroli, patchouli, rose, rosemary

Allergy chamomile, lavender, patchouli

Athlete's foot lavender, lemongrass, myrrh, patchouli, tea tree

Bleeding geranium, lemon

Boils and carbuncles bergamot, chamomile, lavender, lemon, lime, rosemary, tea tree, thyme

Broken capillaries chamomile, cypress, frankincense, lemon, neroli, rose, sandalwood

Bruises chamomile, fennel, geranium, lavender, marjoram

Burns chamomile, eucalyptus, lavender, geranium

Cellulite cypress, fennel, geranium, grapefruit, juniper, lemon, lime, rosemary

Chapped and cracked skin benzoin, myrrh, patchouli, sandalwood, tea tree

Combination skin geranium, lavender, neroli

Cuts eucalyptus, geranium, lavender, lemon, tea tree

Dermatitis benzoin, juniper, lavender, myrrh, patchouli, peppermint, rosemary

Dry skin benzoin, carrot seed, chamomile, clary sage, frankincense, geranium, jasmine, lavender, neroli, rose, sandalwood, vetivert, ylang ylang

Eczema bergamot, geranium, juniper, lavender, myrrh, patchouli, rosemary

Herpes bergamot, eucalyptus, lavender, lemon, tea tree

Inflamed, red, irritated skin benzoin, chamomile, clary sage, geranium, lavender, myrrh, neroli, patchouli, peppermint, rose

Mature skin carrot seed, clary sage, frankincense, geranium, jasmine, lavender, myrrh, neroli, patchouli, rose, sandalwood

Measles (and other infectious diseases) bergamot, eucalyptus, geranium, lemon, lemongrass, rosemary, tea tree

Oily and open pores bergamot, cajeput, clary sage, cypress, frankincense, geranium, juniper, lavender, lemon, lemongrass, lime, mandarin, peppermint, sandalwood, tea tree, ylang ylang

Perspiration cypress, lemongrass, tea tree

Psoriasis benzoin, bergamot, cajeput, chamomile, lavender, tea tree

Scars carrot seed, jasmine, mandarin, neroli, patchouli

Sensitive chamomile, geranium, jasmine, lavender, neroli, rose

Sunburn clary sage, lavender, peppermint

Varicose veins cypress, geranium, ginger, lemon, neroli, tea tree

Warts and verrucae lemon, lime, tea tree

Wounds and sores benzoin, frankincense, geranium, juniper, myrrh, patchouli, tea tree, thyme

Wrinkles carrot seed, clary sage, frankincense, myrrh, patchouli, rose, rosemary

www.ingramcontent.com/pod-product-compliance
Ingram Content Group UK Ltd.
Pitfield, Milton Keynes, MK11 3LW, UK
UKHW021828270225
455667UK00014B/156